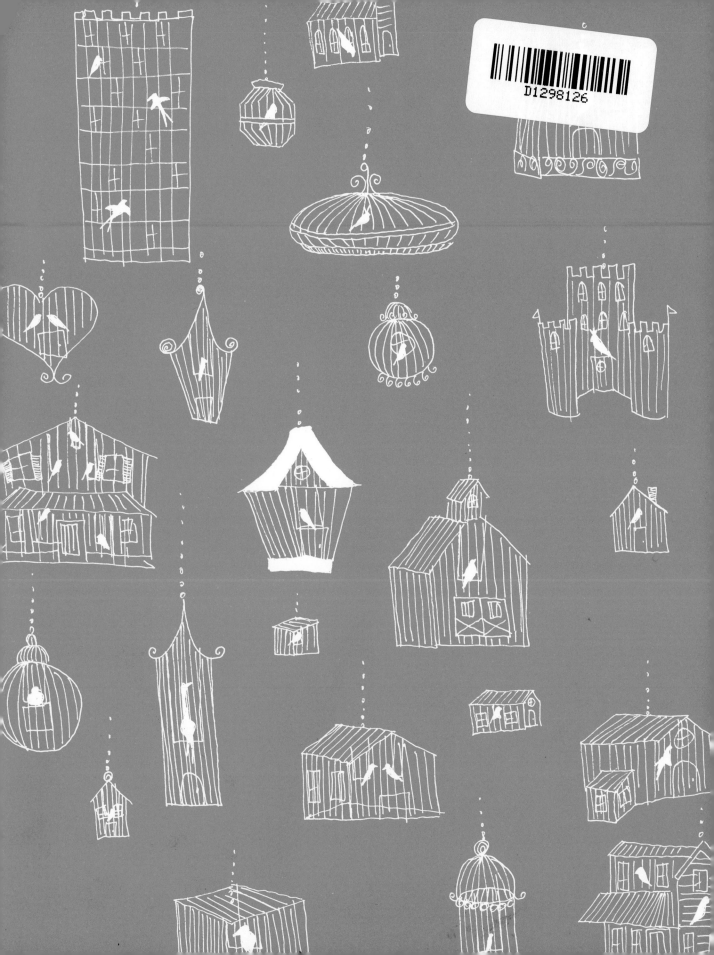

Ruby
and
Bubbles

story and pictures by

Rosie Winstead

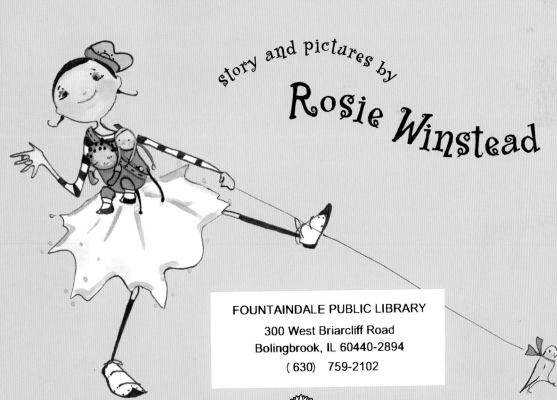

Dial Books for Young Readers

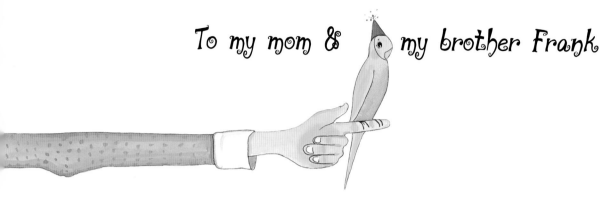

To my mom & my brother Frank

DIAL BOOKS FOR YOUNG READERS

A division of Penguin Young Readers Group · Published by The Penguin Group
Penguin Group (USA) Inc., 375 Hudson Street, New York, NY 10014, U.S.A. ·
Penguin Group (Canada), 90 Eglinton Avenue East, Suite 700, Toronto,
Ontario, Canada M4P 2Y3 (a division of Pearson Penguin Canada Inc.) · Penguin Books Ltd,
80 Strand, London WC2R 0RL, England · Penguin Ireland, 25 St. Stephen's Green,
Dublin 2, Ireland (a division of Penguin Books Ltd) · Penguin Group (Australia),
250 Camberwell Road, Camberwell, Victoria 3124, Australia (a division of Pearson Australia
Group Pty Ltd) · Penguin Books India Pvt Ltd, 11 Community Centre, Panchsheel Park,
New Delhi-110 017, India · Penguin Group (NZ), Cnr Airborne and Rosedale Roads, Albany,
Auckland 1310, New Zealand (a division of Pearson New Zealand Ltd) · Penguin Books (South Africa)
(Pty) Ltd, 24 Sturdee Avenue, Rosebank, Johannesburg 2196, South Africa ·
Penguin Books Ltd, Registered Offices: 80 Strand, London WC2R 0RL, England

Designed by Teresa Kietlinski
Text set in Mrs Eaves Roman
Manufactured in China on acid-free paper

1 3 5 7 9 10 8 6 4 2

Library of Congress Cataloging-in-Publication Data
Winstead, Rosie.
Ruby and Bubbles / story and pictures by Rosie Winstead.
p. cm.
Summary: Ruby discovers how much she means to her pet bird, Bubbles,
when he helps her deal with two bullying girls.
ISBN 0-8037-3024-1
[1. Birds—Fiction. 2. Pets—Fiction. 3. Bullies—Fiction. 4. Friendship—Fiction.] I. Title.
PZ7.W7526Ru 2006

[E]—dc22   2004015310

The art was created using watercolors, pencil, pen, and ink.

Once upon a time, long, long ago, Ruby was little.

But now she is big,

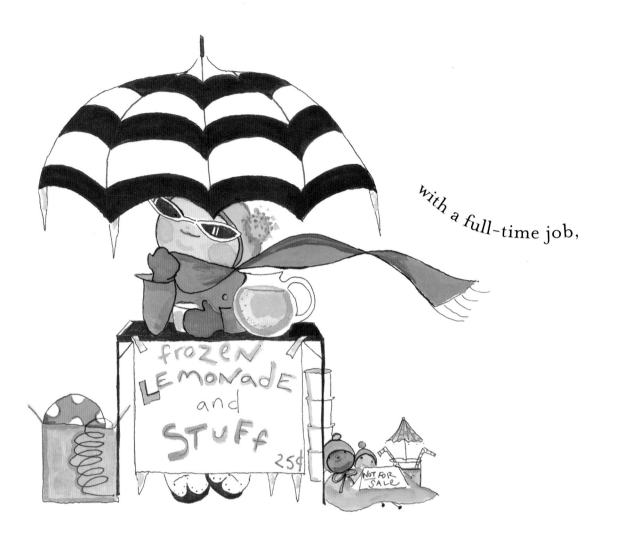

with a full-time job,

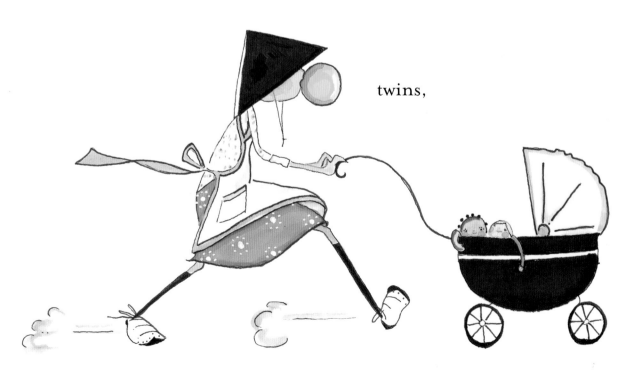

twins,

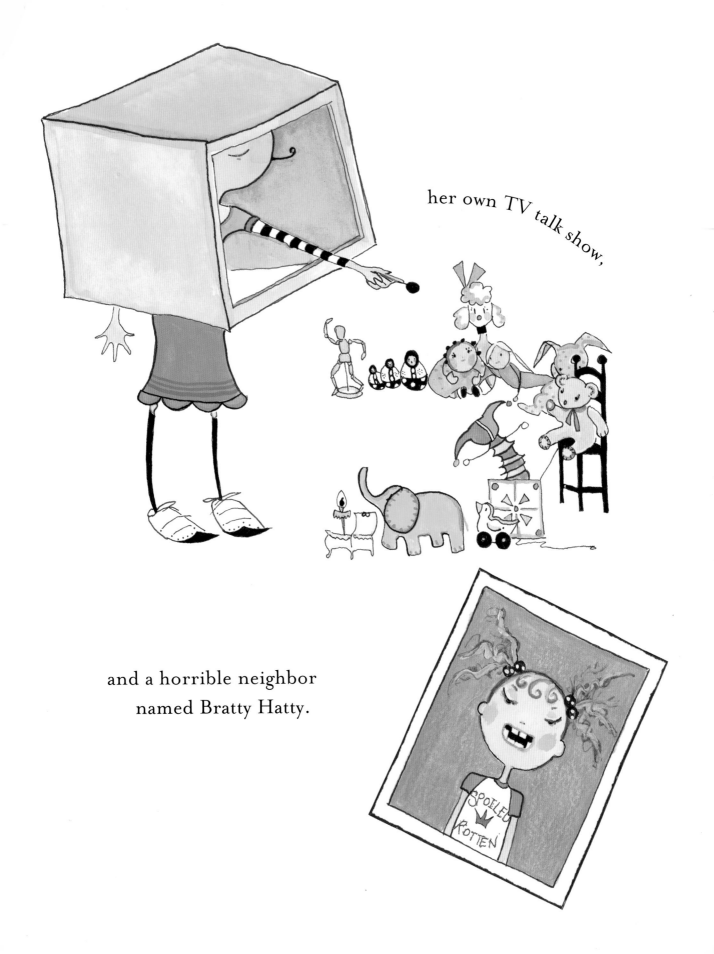

her own TV talk show,

and a horrible neighbor
named Bratty Hatty.

One day when Ruby was working, Hatty and her best friend, Mean Maureen, came by.

"Nobody to play with, Ruby-dooby?" sneered Bratty Hatty. "Me and Maureen are going to give each other total makeovers!"

"It's just us!" said Mean Maureen. "And you totally can't come!"

Ruby didn't even *want* to play with those awful girls.

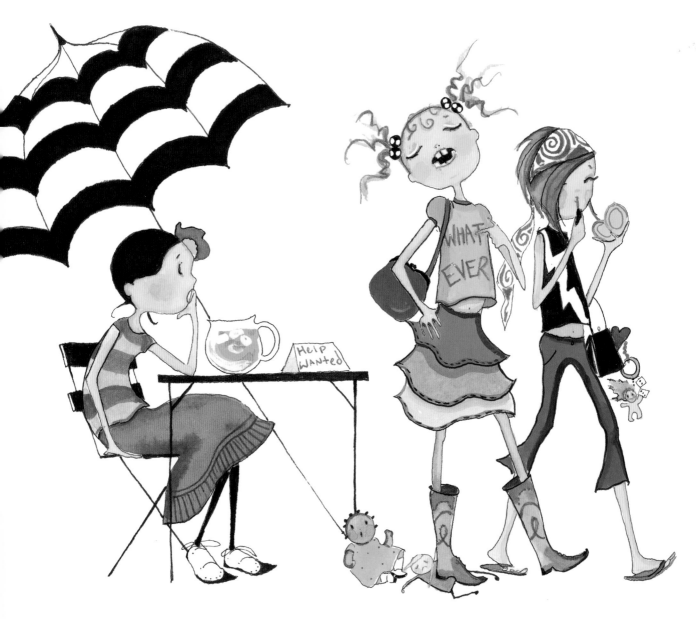

But it had been a long morning,
and she was ready for a break.

So Ruby decided to take the rest
of the day off,

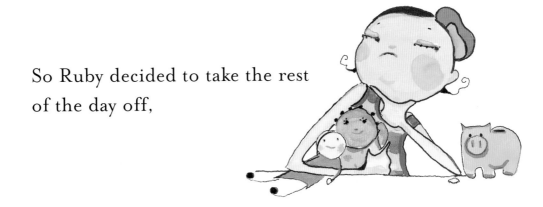

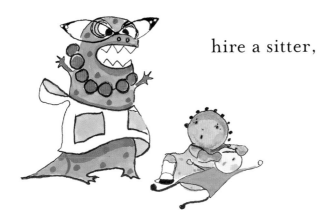

hire a sitter,

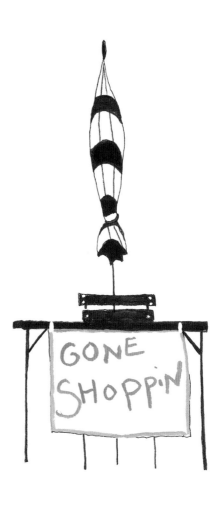

and do what she liked best.

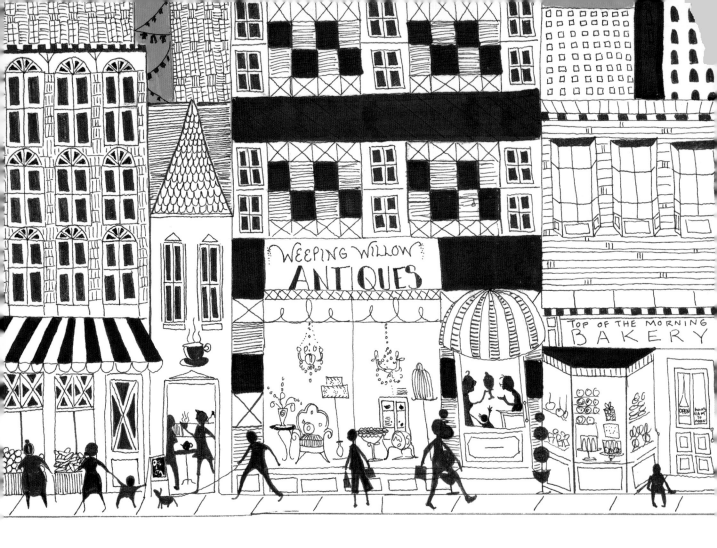

After one lolly-ring, a candy necklace,
and three gum balls, Ruby was ready
to head back home, when . . .
something caught her eye.

It was cute, yellow, and just her size.
Ruby walked in with a dream,

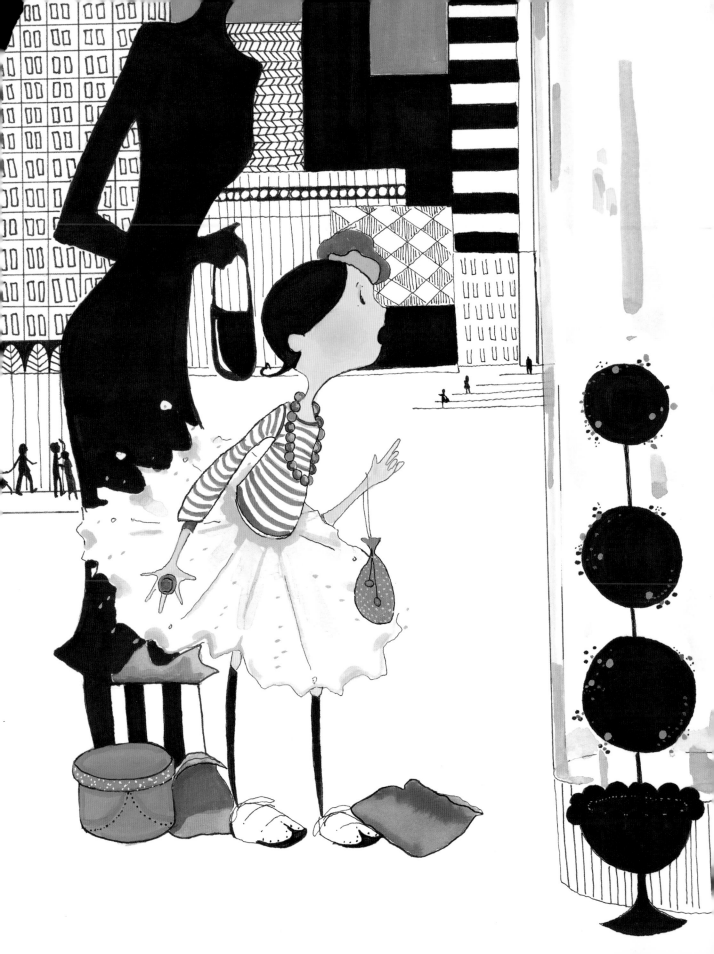

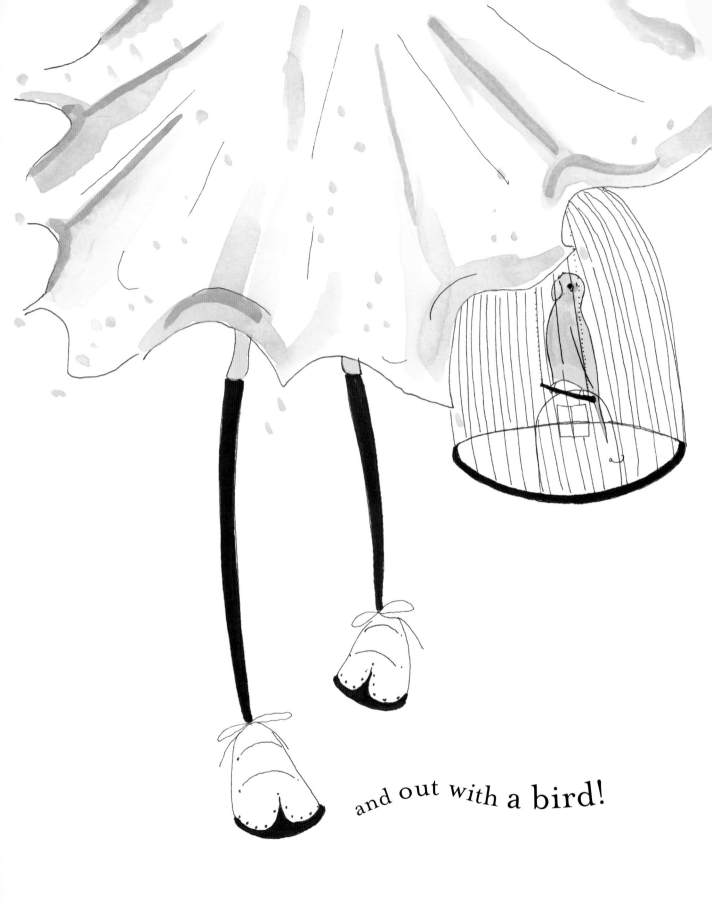

and out with a bird!

What could Ruby name him?
"Jimmy? Nah!

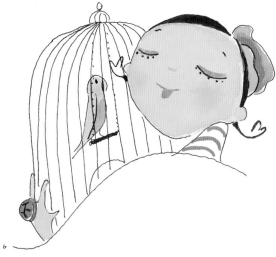

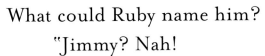

"Chirpadoodlehead? Too long.

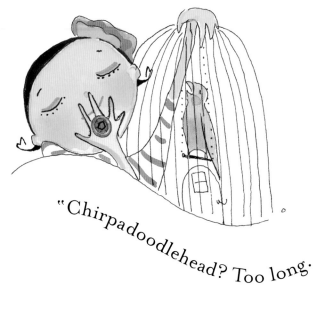

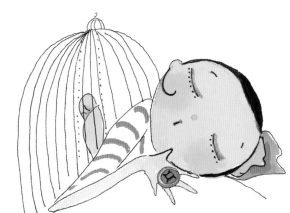

"Birdie?
How bor-ing!"

Ruby thought
and chewed
and . . .
POP

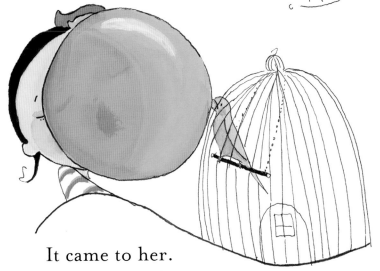

It came to her.
"*Bubbles!* Yeah, Bubbles!" So Bubbles it was.

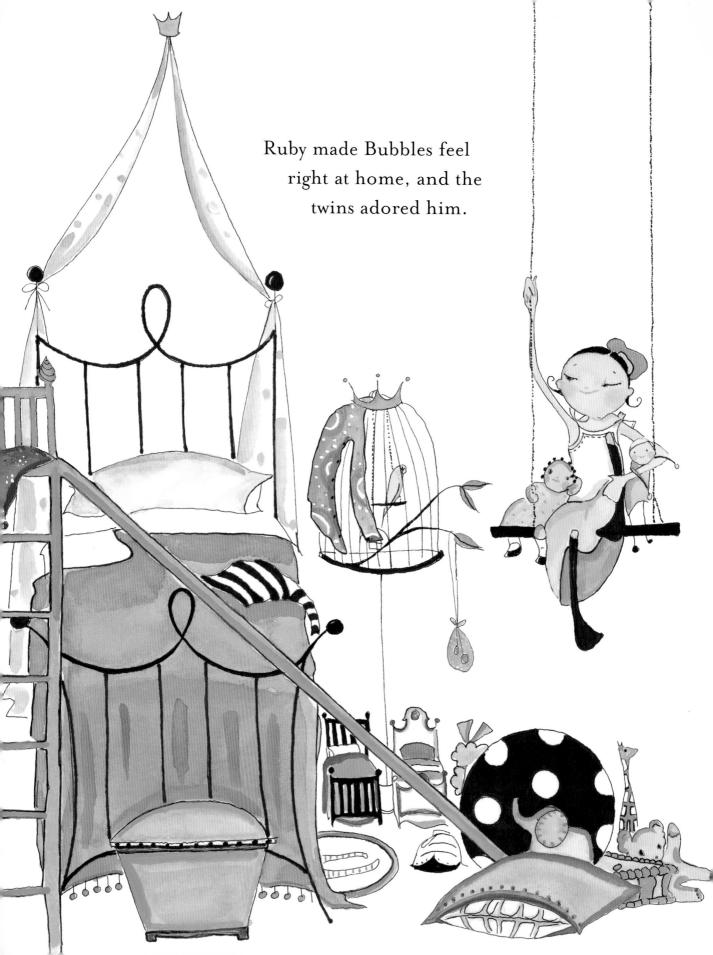

Ruby made Bubbles feel
right at home, and the
twins adored him.

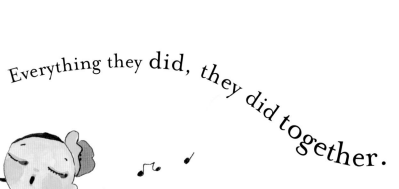

Everything they **did**, they did together.

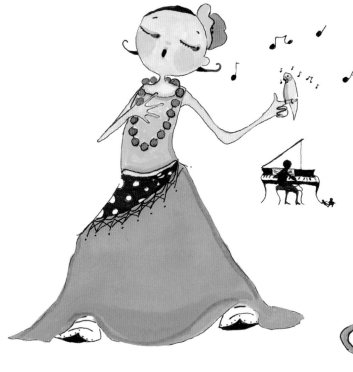

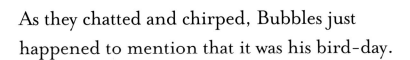

As they chatted and chirped, Bubbles just
happened to mention that it was his bird-day.

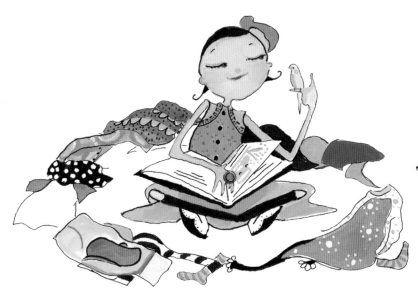

"You know what?"
Ruby told Bubbles.
"I'm going to throw you
a **bird-day** party!"

Everyone was invited, even Mean Maureen and Bratty Hatty.
(Ruby's mom made her.)
Ruby wanted everything to be extra-shiny and pretty
for the party. The twins helped. A little.

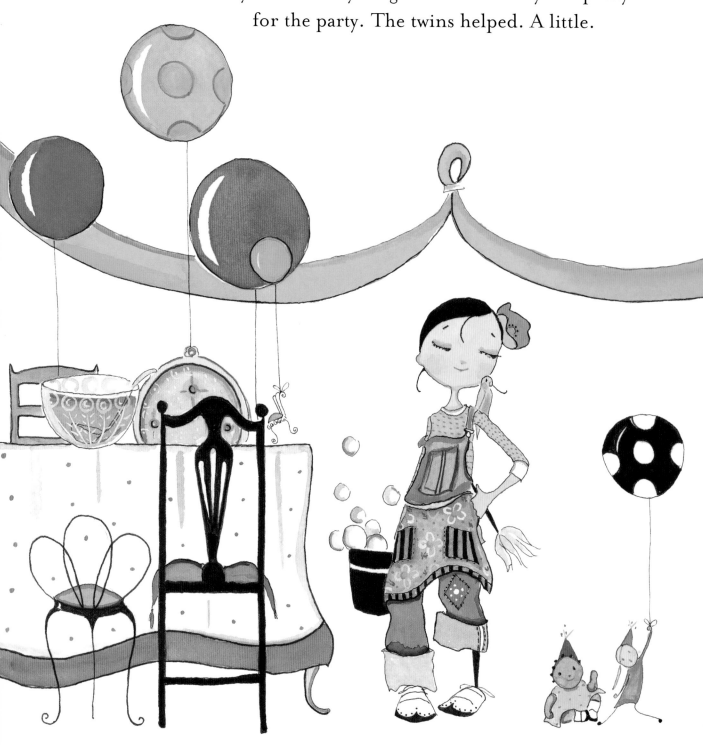

"This is my very best friend, Bubbles!" Ruby told all of her guests.
And everyone seemed to love him . . .
well, almost everyone.

"That's not a friend, that's a bird!" Hatty shouted.

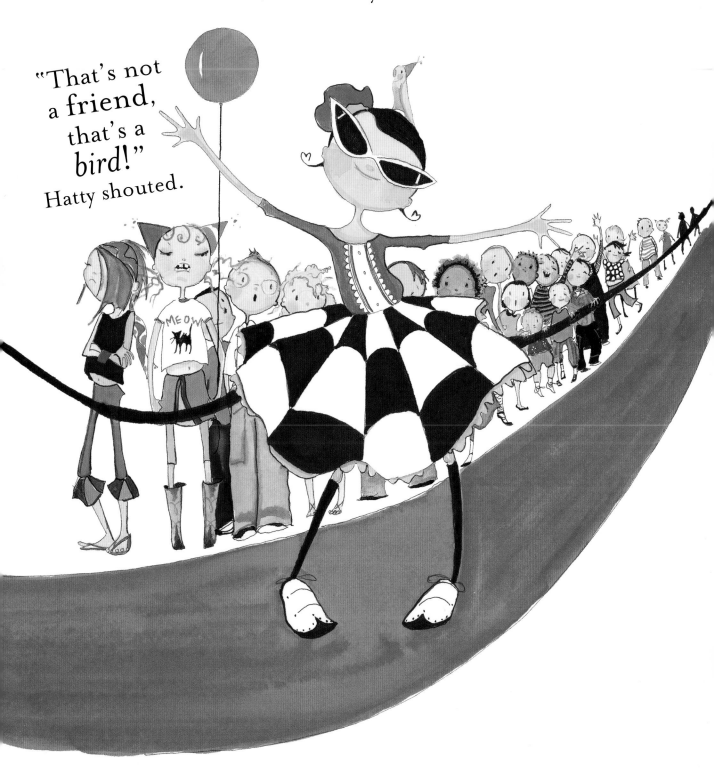

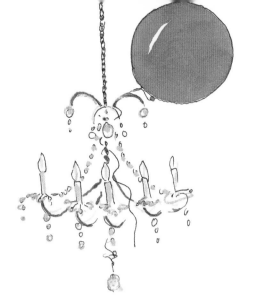

Hatty untied the balloon
from her wrist.

"Go on, Bubble-head!
Go get my balloon!"
she shrieked.

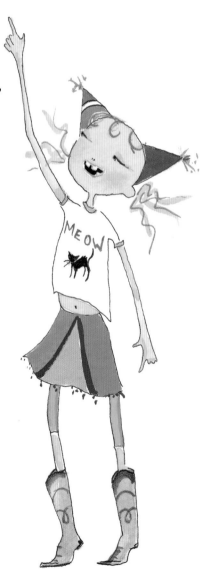

But
Bubbles
wouldn't.

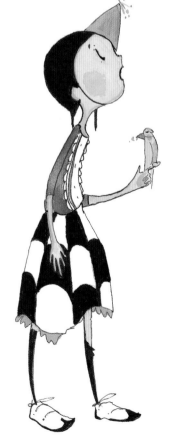

"He's not even a real bird, he can't fly!"
chimed Mean Maureen.

"Ruby's a bird-brain!" said Hatty.

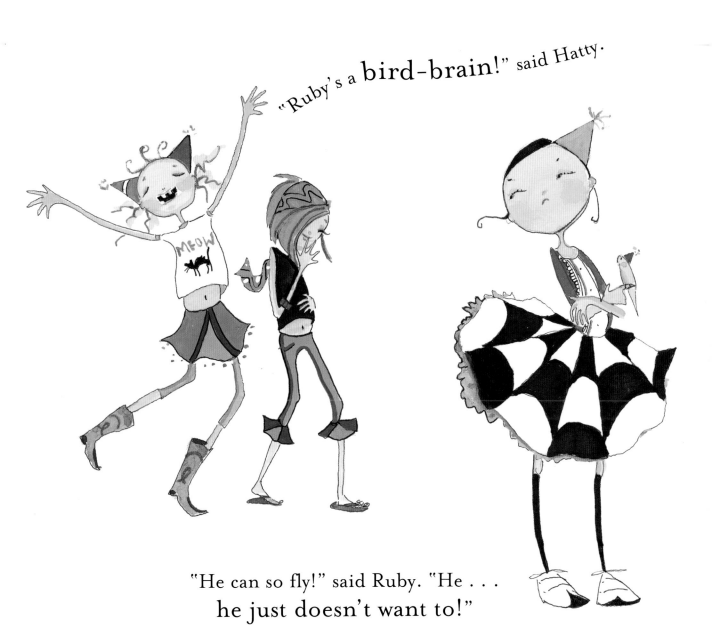

"He can so fly!" said Ruby. "He . . .
he just doesn't want to!"

"Bird-brain, bird-brain, Ruby-dooby, Dooby-do,"

chanted Hatty and Maureen as they flapped around the party. Some of the other kids even joined in.

After that the party ended quickly. "Sorry, Ruby," said Sweet Pete. "Your bird, umm, friend seems nice. Even if he doesn't fly."

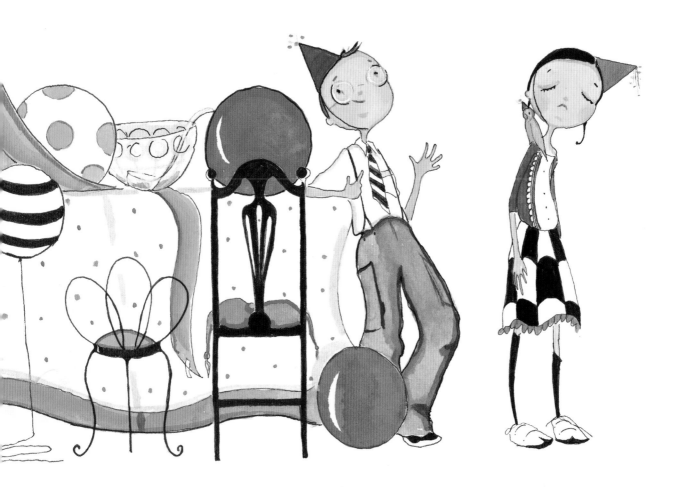

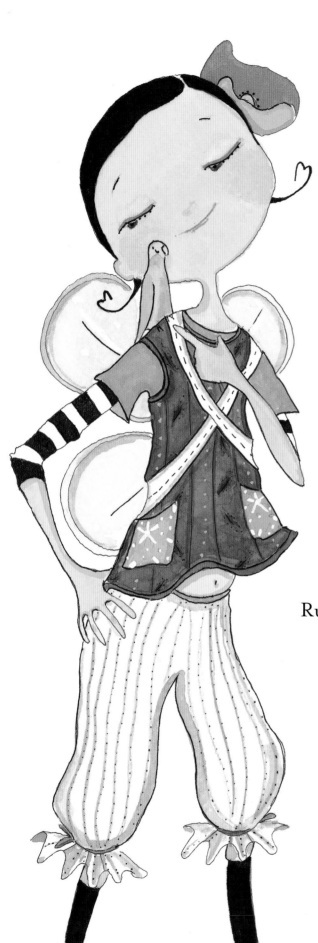

The next day,
Ruby decided to teach Bubbles to fly.
Ms. Ruby would be his teacher.

"Maybe you just need more feathers?"
asked Ruby.

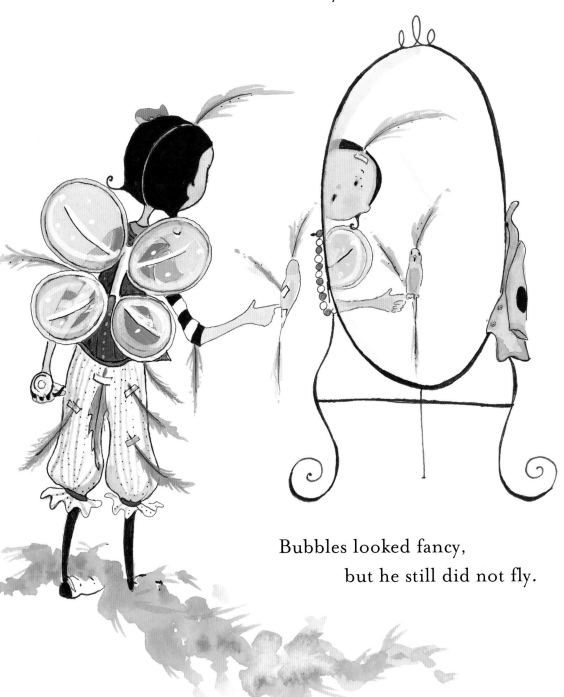

Bubbles looked fancy,
but he still did not fly.

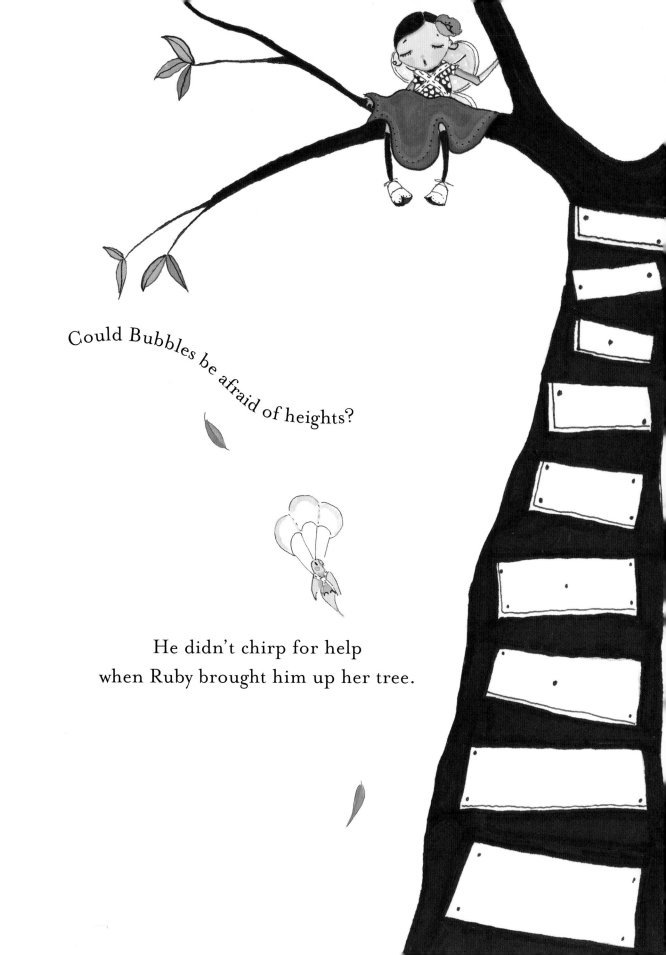

Could Bubbles be afraid of heights?

He didn't chirp for help
when Ruby brought him up her tree.

"Maybe you need to build up your wing muscles?"
Ruby wondered. But the workout didn't work out.

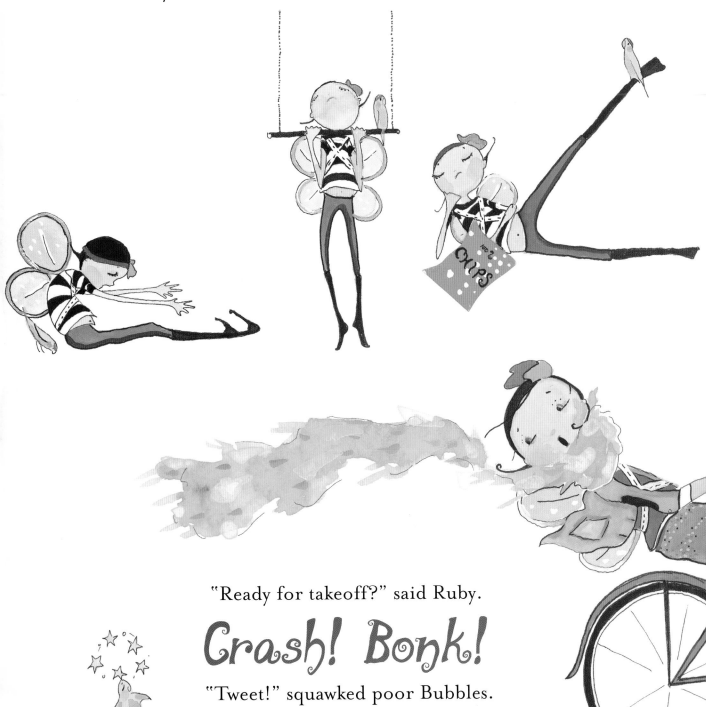

"Ready for takeoff?" said Ruby.

Crash! Bonk!

"Tweet!" squawked poor Bubbles.

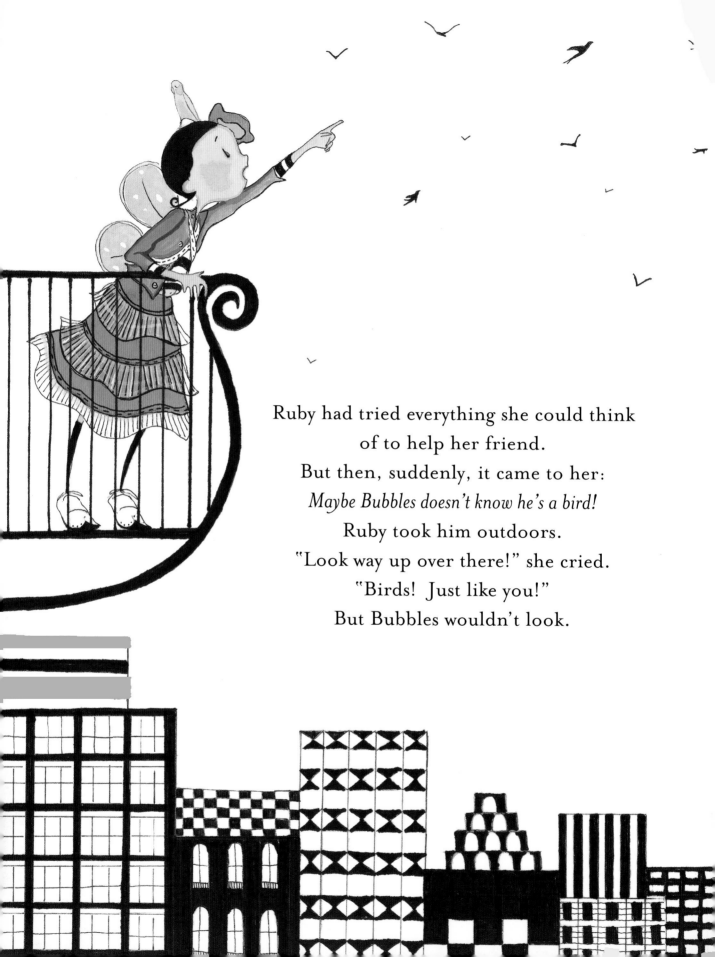

Ruby had tried everything she could think
of to help her friend.
But then, suddenly, it came to her:
Maybe Bubbles doesn't know he's a bird!
Ruby took him outdoors.
"Look way up over there!" she cried.
"Birds! Just like you!"
But Bubbles wouldn't look.

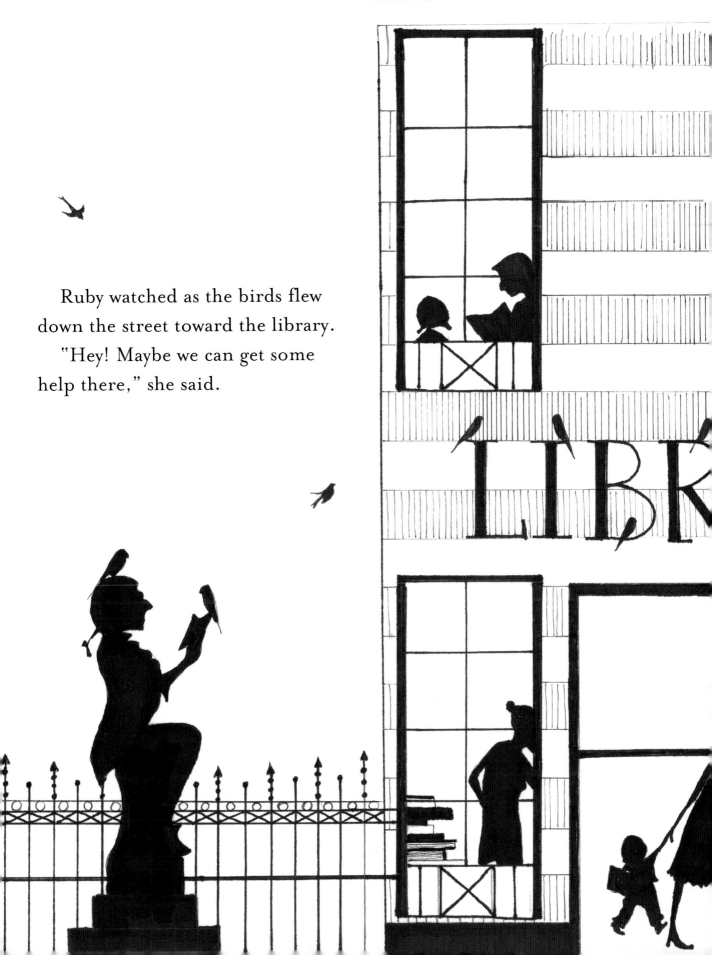

Ruby watched as the birds flew
down the street toward the library.
"Hey! Maybe we can get some
help there," she said.

After taking a look at a few books . . .

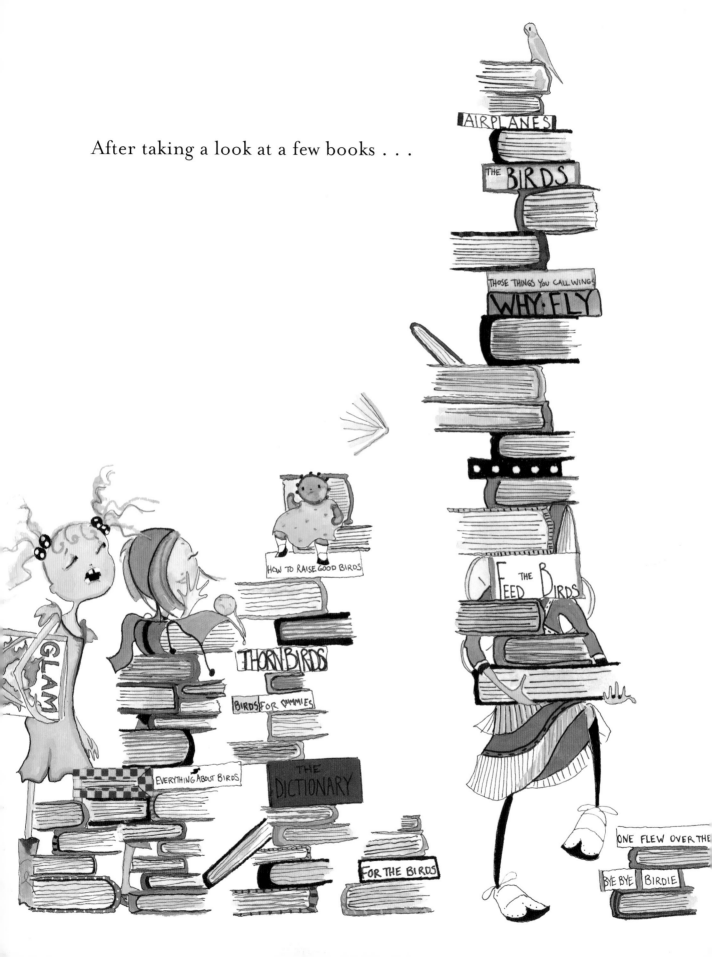

AIRPLANES

THE BIRDS

THOSE THINGS YOU CALL WINGS

WHY·FLY

FEED THE BIRDS

HOW TO RAISE GOOD BIRDS

GLAM

THORNBIRDS

BIRDS FOR DUMMIES

EVERYTHING ABOUT BIRDS

THE DICTIONARY

FOR THE BIRDS

ONE FLEW OVER THE

BYE BYE BIRDIE

Ruby realized that Bubbles wasn't the only odd bird walking around.

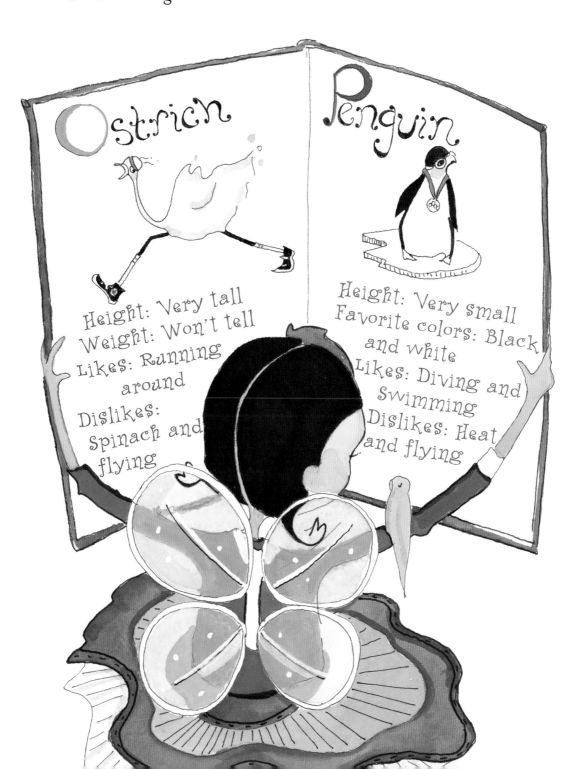

Ostrich

Height: Very tall
Weight: Won't tell
Likes: Running around
Dislikes: Spinach and flying

Penguin

Height: Very small
Favorite colors: Black and white
Likes: Diving and Swimming
Dislikes: Heat and flying

They started to head back home, when . . .

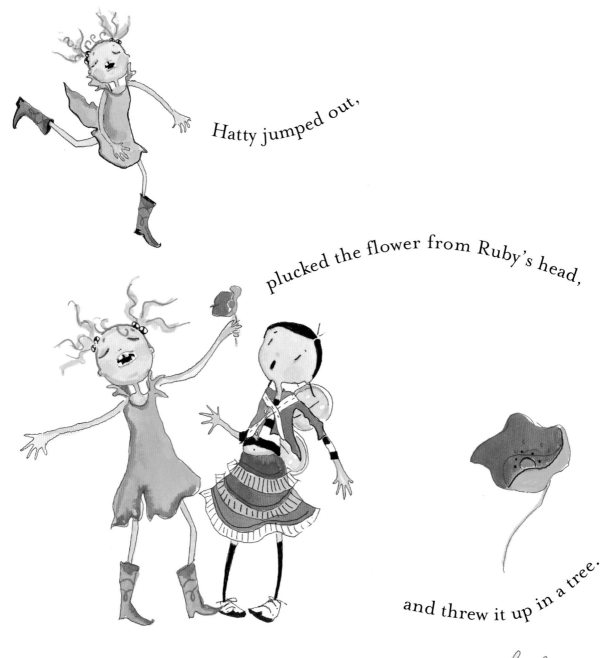

Hatty jumped out,

plucked the flower from Ruby's head,

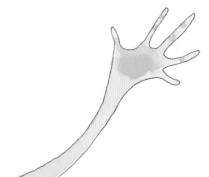

and threw it up in a tree.

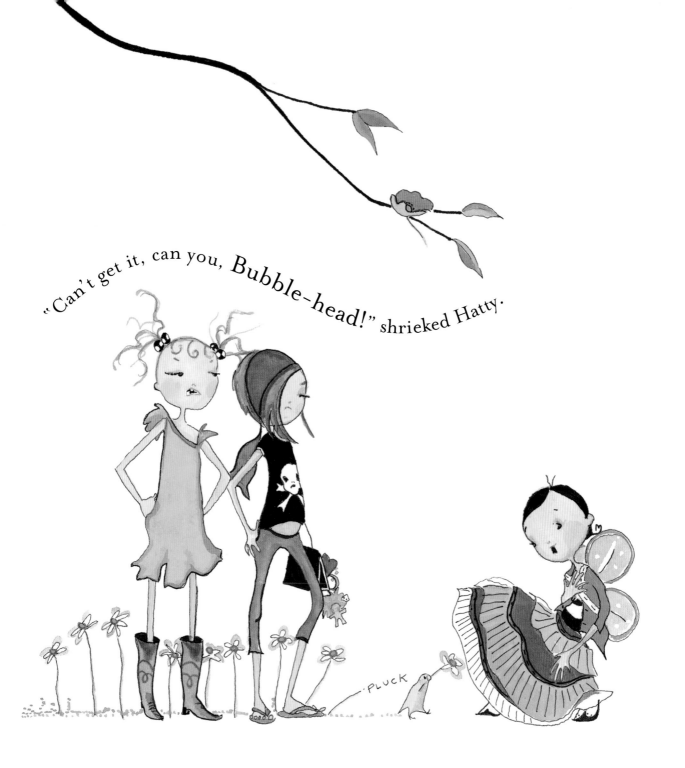

"Can't get it, can you, Bubble-head!" shrieked Hatty.

But Bubbles knew just what to do.
He just picked the prettiest flower he could find . . .
for his Ruby.

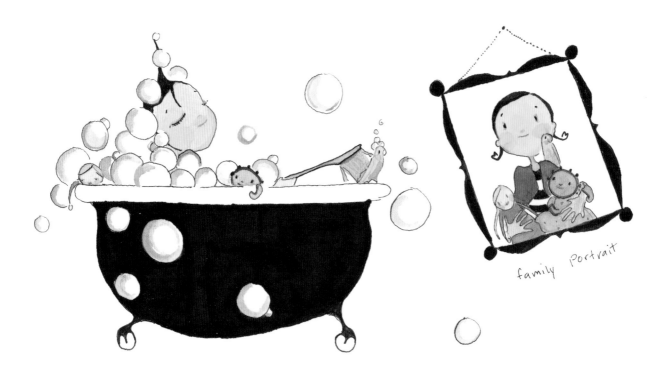

family portrait

Bubbles never did fly.
But Ruby knew it didn't matter. After all . . .
Bubbles could always catch a ride with his best friend.

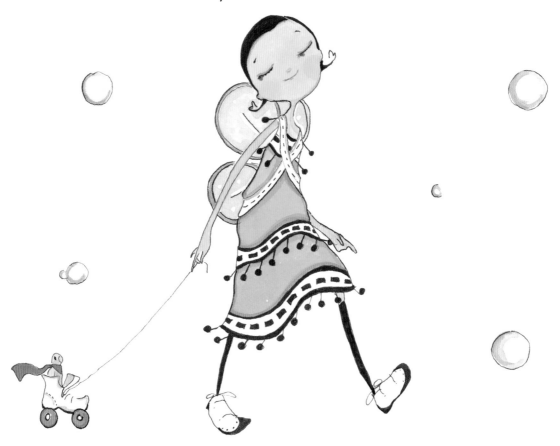

As for Bratty Hatty and Mean Maureen,

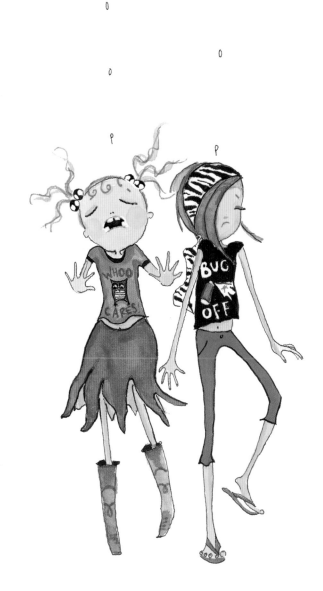

they stayed bratty and mean . . . until some flying birds
dropped them a little lesson.

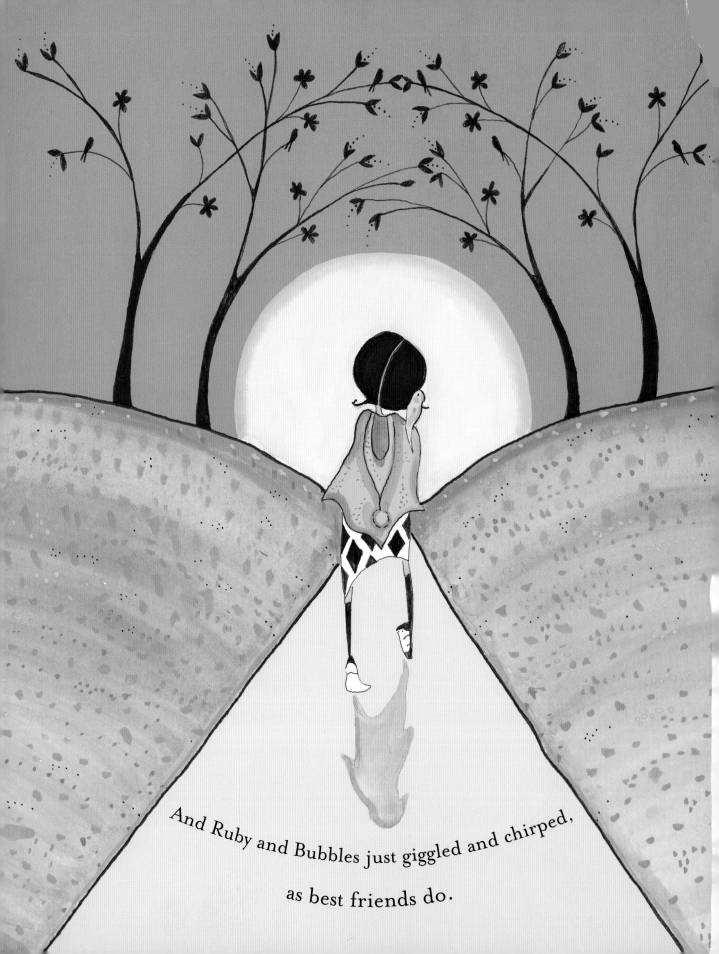

And Ruby and Bubbles just giggled and chirped,

as best friends do.

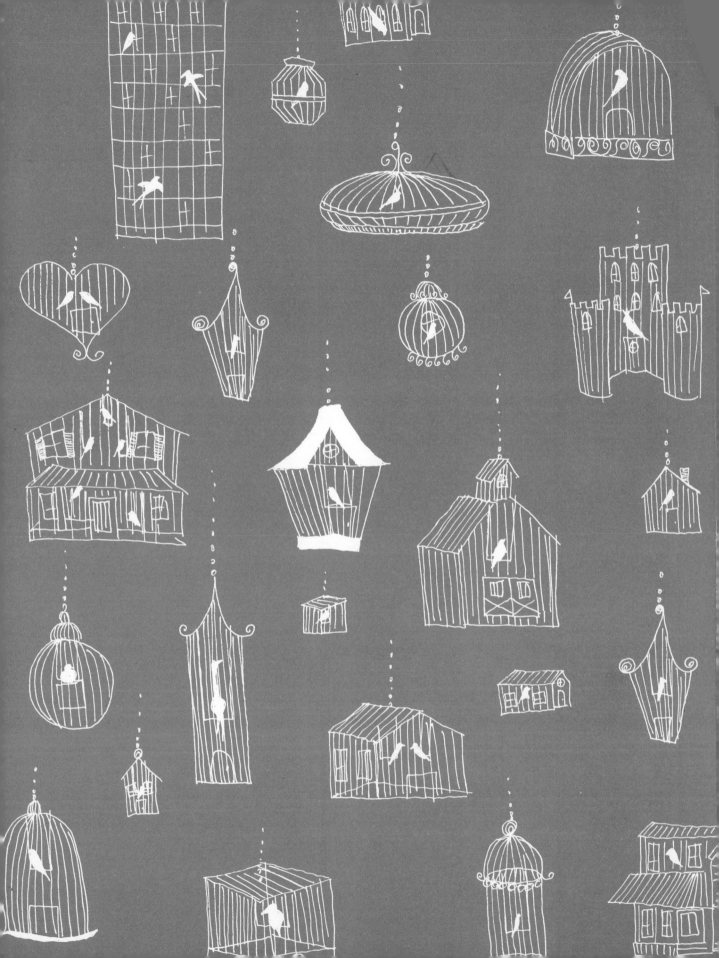